MW00914851

Healthy Habits

30 Healthy Habits and 30 Amazing No Gym Needed Workouts That Will Help You Lose Weight, Remove Negative Thinking and Minimize Stress!

John Mayo

MY FREE GIFT TO YOU:

Learn 14 phenomenal smoothie recipes and lifestyle hacks that will boost your productivity and revitalize your body! This book has helped thousands of people, and you're next!

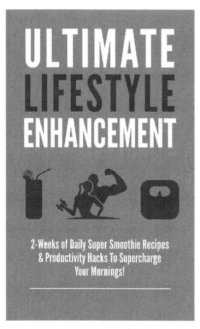

The above book is a gift, given to you as a sincere thank you for purchasing this book. I hope it helps you increase the quality of your life. Download this FREE book by typing in the below link:
https://zenithpublishing.leadpages.net/lifestyle-enhancement/

Enjoy!

Table of Contents:

HEALTHY HABITS

Chapter 1- Introduction:

Fitness is a word that has been more abused than fast food over the last ten years. It seems like every day there is a new YouTube fitness sensation or infomercial channel trying to sell you something that will make you fit quickly and with minimal effort. I'm sick of overweight, cigarette smoking doctors preaching the importance of good health to everybody that walks into their office. I've only seen two healthy looking doctors in my life and that seems quite ironic to me.

I once said "I'd rather be moderately fit, than extremely strong" and I still stand beside that statement, even though most of my friends thought it was stupid. As a 24 year old male, discrediting strength in any way is a sure-fire way to look weak in front of other guys. The truth of the matter is that strength is only one of many dimensions of fitness. By being a well-rounded fit person, strength is implied. Would you rather eat a big plate full of only steak, or have a modest portion of steak and indulge in the rest of the buffet?

I define fitness as a 'general sense of well being stemming from a multitude of different factors including, but not limited to, physical activeness, body image, coordination, diet, sleep schedule and mental stimulation.' This sounds like a lot and it is, which is why increasing fitness takes way more than a piece of workout equipment, a five minute per day circuit, or some kind of 'super supplement.' That is lesson number one: fitness is not an easy thing to achieve; it is something that should be striven for. If it were easy there would be a lot more fit people in the world, but it takes consistent effort and it is this effort that makes it worth it in the end.

As I write this I am on a two-month road trip around the United States and I feel awful, even though I'm having an amazing time, with fantastic people. Why do I feel awful you ask? Because my fitness level has decreased dramatically since I left Canada. When you leave your regular life and restrict yourself to the confines of a small vehicle it becomes relatively easy to isolate factors that are affecting your personal happiness. My physical activity has plummeted, my flexibility (or lack thereof) has gone down the drain, my diet consists of mostly canned food/ gas station meals and my sleep schedule is a train wreck. Before I willingly crammed myself into this small Mitsubishi, I felt amazing. I was active every day, eating well, sleeping great and having lots of sex.

Fitness should not be viewed as a quick fad that you achieve and then have forever. It is a lifestyle that needs to be maintained regularly, just like a car. Don't let yourself become one of those people who care more about what they're putting in their car, than what they're putting in their own bodies, or you're sure to break down regularly. If you really think about it, your body is one big complex machine and if you're not particular about how you're fuelling and running it, then you are destined to crash and burn.

My name is John Mayo, I'm not very flexible, I sleep decently, eat horrible food a couple times a week, drink alcohol on occasion, have sex as much as possible and I consider myself fairly fit. I'm not writing this in an attempt to stroke my ego; I'm just an average guy who likes to feel good as much as I can. I got into fitness as a young age as a flat-water kayaker and experienced success in the sport for the seven years that I competed. I became a national champion in two events and got to travel to the United States and Europe to compete.

When I quit kayaking due to a back injury I became very paranoid about falling out of shape. This paranoia stemmed from the fact that I was going from a structured daily training regiment, to absolutely nothing. Sport and fitness were all I had known growing up, so once university started I began hitting the gym solo for the first time in my life. I started developing my own workout plans and really began to enjoy myself. I liked the idea of engineering my own fitness and being able to push myself without a coach.

I'm going to show you how to throw an axe in your daily rituals and change things up so that you can revolutionize your life! Yes, there is a woman on the cover of this book. Yes I am a man writing this book, but do not be fooled, the tips and tricks in this book are useful for both sexes (or anybody in between). Now, if you have been following me and my other books you will realize that I know a thing or two about feeling good, feeling fit, thinking positively and living stress free. I do not claim to be some enlightened guru who spends his time slowly roaming the beaches at 5 in the morning. No, I am merely a regular individual who has taken control of his mind and his circumstances and attempted to fully optimize his life. My primary goal is to help you do the same.

I love helping people change their lives and watching people succeed and flourish brings me unprecedented joy. Sometimes as I walk through the grocery store and I see someone that looks upset or depressed with their life I just want to reach out to them, right then and there and say:

"If you want help, if you want to become happier, I am here to help you"

I am not exactly sure how people would take that. Some would probably accept my help and ask me to teach them how to revolutionize their life and some would probably punch me in the face and tell me that they are already happy. Please do not think that I am writing this book in a self-righteous way. I would never use the words cocky and conceded to describe my personality traits, and I do not think my friends and peers would either.

I have organized this book in the most simplistic way that I could. The primary purpose of this book is to disclose some of the things that I think can lead you to a life of increased fitness and better health. While there is some external research cited, most of the writing here is my opinion/ personal experiences and things that work for me. There are 8 aspects of fitness that I believe people can improve upon to make themselves happier. These 8 aspects are; diet, sleep, flexibility, cardio, core, functional strength, sex and mental sharpness. I will provide only information that I deem to be useful in order to keep things concise. Keep in mind; once you habitually do something, even something painful or difficult, it becomes extraordinarily simple

I will then go from 1 to 30 and break down the 30 daily habits will help you lose weight, remove negative thinking and minimize stress. After covering all of the habits I will provide you with 30 fantastic workouts that you can do from the comfort of your own home. I recommend doing one of these workouts per day for an entire month to see what results you can get! I hope you can use this book as a tool to better your life because that is my ultimate intention here.

Life is all about getting into routines, routines that will empower, inspire, energize and enhance your existence. If you can incorporate the following habits, information and workouts into your daily routine, I challenge you to not feel like a more uplifted person. Good luck and enjoy the book.

Chapter 2- Diet:

If you eat like crap, you will feel like crap. This is the most basic yet true statement in the fitness world. If you're going to ignore your eating habits completely and strictly focus on exercise, don't bother reading any further. If you want a great physique you need to eat well, period. Modern society is not designed to aid you in your quest of healthy eating; it is designed to make things that are cheap and convenient for you so that you buy lots. I recently looked up McDonalds health facts; we all know that this sad excuse for a restaurant is bad, but did you know the double quarter pounder meal has almost 3 grams of trans fat? That should be illegal but its not, why? Because McDonalds is a billion dollar, genius company that knows how to make people buy shitty food for the sake of convenience. The bottom line here is that you need to take responsibility for your own diet.

Do not read the word diet and think 'temporary.' Show me someone on a temporary diet and I'll show you someone who will soon be eating like crap again. Your diet should be your lifestyle. Make eating well a lifetime habit and not a two-week fad.

Since there is no universally agreed upon 'perfect diet' I will provide a brief summary of my diet and the rules I try to follow.

-What I Try to Avoid:

Fried foods, white rice, bread, potatoes, cereal, beer/ liquid carbs, fatty sauces, trans fats (obviously), high fructose corn syrup (glucose- fructose in Canada).

* I consume every single thing listed above; I just try to consume very minimal amounts of each.

-What I Typically Try to Eat:

Quinoa & quinoa pasta, whole grain or multigrain bread (if I eat bread at all), avocadoes, kale, spinach, max 2-3 eggs a day, brown rice, ground flaxseed (frozen or refrigerated), chia seeds (great mixed with water), chicken breast, ground tomatoes (substitute for pasta sauce), bananas, natural peanut/ almond butter, dates, unsalted nuts and almonds, black beans, cliff bars, mixed vegetables, unsweetened almond milk, unsweetened coconut water/ oil, LOTS AND LOTS OF WATER!

-Here is what I would consider a good day of eating for myself.

Breakfast:

Large smoothie consisting of 2 bananas, 2 dates, 1 tbs of natural peanut butter, 1 handful of kale and spinach, 1 tbs of ground flaxseed, 1 tbs of chia seeds, 1 tbs of coconut oil, lots of cinnamon, 1 handful of assorted frozen fruit, unsweetened almond milk and coconut water (add until there's a sufficient amount of liquid in the smoothie.

Lunch:

Burrito made with whole-wheat pita, avocado, black beans, quinoa/ brown rice, tomatoes, tuna, and sweet potato.

Snack:

Cliff bar, carrots and broccoli.

Dinner:

Chicken quinoa with natural tomato sauce (crushed tomatoes), spinach salad with some light vinaigrette dressing

As you can see, my breakfast packs a punch and I fit as many things as I can into my smoothie. With my smoothies I also take 1000 IU of vitamin D, multivitamin, fish oil, and 1200 mcg of vitamin B12. It's especially important to stay hydrated during the day if you are staying active and sweating. Every time I pass a water fountain I take a drink and I always try to keep a water bottle with me.

Once a week however, I have a cheat day and I spike my caloric intake by eating whatever I want. This is not a bad thing and it will allow you to maintain a healthy diet throughout the week. Sometimes if I find I can't wait for one specific day, I will have a couple of cheat meals during the week instead. If 90% of what you're eating is healthy then you're allowed to slip up sometimes. Keep in mind that I am not a nutritionist or a dietician. This is simply what I tend to eat/ avoid and it works very well for me and I feel awesome when I follow the above guidelines.

Chapter 3- Sleep:

Sleep is obviously a crucial factor when it comes to your energy level. Most people solemnly believe that 8 hours is the universally prescribed sleep duration. Dean Karnazses is a living rebuttal of the 8-hour claim. Karnzases decided that he was wasting too much time sleeping so he began sleeping 4 hours a night. This seems to be working for him because he regularly competes in ultra marathons and he once ran 50 consecutive marathons, in all 50 of the United States, in 50 days, all on 4 hours of sleep per night. This guy is obviously a freak of nature when it comes to running, but could he be on to something when it comes to sleep cycles?

I don't claim to sleep 4 hours a night; I usually get between 6 and 7 hours, sometimes with a 20-minute nap during the day. Tim Ferris did extensive research on polyphasic sleep (Sleeping multiple times within 24 hours) in "The 4 Hour Body." Ferris essentially found that for every 1.5 hours of core sleep you subtract, you can still feel just as energized if you add a twenty minute nap during the day for every 1.5 hours lost. These naps should be strict and as close to twenty minutes as you can possibly get. I personally find Ferris' model to work but only to an extent. Once you dip below 3 hours of core sleep and 3 twenty-minute naps, things begin to get a little iffy. I do not know anybody who has time for 5 or 6 naps during the day and I found it impossible to stay energized running on anything less than 3 hours of core sleep. Even 3 hours with 3 naps sometimes left me feeling exhausted.

One thing Ferris definitely gets wrong in his book is sleep position. He claims that sleeping on your stomach; in an immobilizing half military crawl position, is the best way to sleep. If you don't have a spine or your immune to back pain then this position might work for you. Otherwise you should sleep on your back with pillow(s) under your knees, or you could do your back an even bigger favor and sleep on your side, with one pillow between your legs, one under your head and one under the arm that's on top. I try to use the latter sleeping position as much as possible, especially since I injured my back a few years ago. Every chiropractor, physiotherapist and Osteopath I went to recommended this position and I have to say it works very well.

I would advise you to question the 8-hour sleep model and play around with different core sleep and nap schedules. Everybody is different and you need to find out what works best for you. You might find that you can give yourself more productive time in exchange for less sleep, all while maintaining similar or higher energy levels. I try not to eat within an hour of going to sleep to avoid putting on pointless weight and I try to stick to a consistent sleeping position and schedule as much as possible.

Chapter 4- Core:

This is my absolute favorite part of working out. Prepare yourself for some core workouts from hell as you continue to read this book. The core is the essence of your entire body and if your core is weak, you are weak. Keep in mind that your core is more than just your abs; it is the stabilization system of your entire body. Your core is basically every part of your body that is not your head, arms or legs. I find that when I'm working my core a lot, my general workout techniques tend to improve, I feel more balanced and I'm way less likely to get an injury. I work my core at least 3 times a week and the stronger my core gets, the more I enjoy the gym.

Doing ab workouts is not going to get you a six-pack, unless you eat well and have no belly fat. If you have an awful diet and a lot of belly fat, it doesn't matter how hard you work your abs because the fat will be covering up the results. You have to burn that fat off by doing intense core and cardiovascular endurance workouts. This is why you will notice that a lot of the workouts I provide for you will involve running, or they will have no rest, meaning you get a great cardiovascular workout.

If your wondering if a strong core means a nice chiselled six-pack, the answer is: *usually*. Not everyone who has an extremely strong core gets to enjoy the benefits of toned abs. If your core is strong, your cardiovascular capacity is good and you still have belly fat covering your abs, chances are good that your diet sucks. Getting abs is a combination of diet, core exercise and cardio. See the preview for my book "How to Get Abs" at the end of this book for more information about targeting your abdominal region.

Chapter 5- Flexibility:

This is my weakest area of fitness, so I write this chapter as someone trying to gain better flexibility by experimenting with new techniques. I remember being forced to stretch in gym class throughout school when I was younger and hating every second of it. Most people, when they are young, are so flexible that they don't care about maintaining that same level of flexibility. I used to be flexible, then I competed as a kayaker for 7 years, not stretching nearly enough, and now I am as inflexible as a rusty robot.

My downfall was not doing post-workout stretching. I almost never stretched after I had done either a vigorous kayaking or weight workout. I would just leave the paddling club with super tense muscles, head home and go to sleep. Years of this routine have certainly taken a toll on me and I've faced my fair share of injuries because of it.

Since incorporating proper warm-ups before my workouts and at least 15 minutes of post- workout stretching into my routine, I have yet to get an injury. I used to stretch before my workouts but now I only stretch afterwards. This is because I was getting injured about once a year from lifting weights. Two sports therapists suggested that I switch my stretching to after my workout and do dynamic warm-ups at the beginning of workouts. I took this advice and it has been working very well for me.

Here are some good dynamic warm-ups:

Warm-up A) 5- 10 minutes of skipping, 20 lunges

Warm-up B) 30 arms circles (15 each way), 5 burpees, 20 squats, 20 jumping jacks.

Warm-up C) 2 X 30 reps of: jumping jacks, high knees, seal jacks.

These don't have to be difficult, just something to get you moving before your main workout. After your main workout you should stretch for 15- 20 minutes. Not only will this aid your worked muscles in recovering, but you will be less sore the next day as well. Daily stretching sessions will increase flexibility tremendously and decrease the likelihood of getting injured in the gym.

I have sometimes entered the gym feeling slow, weak and sluggish and cancelled my workouts in order to stretch for 40 minutes. On these days I always leave the gym feeling much better than I did coming in. If you come to the realization that you're too tired to get anything out of a scheduled workout, don't feel bad about stretching instead because this is still productive in the long run. I give myself one day completely off in my workout schedule, so I try to stretch lots on that day as well. Look online to find some great stretches for different muscles, create a stretching routine and stick to it everyday. I try to hold every single stretch I do for at least thirty seconds. If you stretch every day for two weeks you will definitely notice an increase in flexibility. Make sure you don't over stretch though; I do about 18 different stretches for thirty seconds each and that's it.

Another way I was able to dramatically increase my flexibility was participating in Brazillian Jiu Jitsu. This low impact martial art forces you to become flexible in order to survive. You're forced to contort your body in many different ways in order to not tap out and lose matches. Two or three weeks of hard jiu jitsu training and you're sure to notice a difference in flexibility. Flexibility isn't the only benefit of jiu jitsu, it's also an amazing full-body workout and you will learn things like how to control your breathing, how to channel your anger, applicable self-defence skills, and how to keep your ego in check.

Last but not least, yoga is an amazing way to improve your flexibility and calm your mind. I love doing yoga at least a few times a week to ground myself and relax my body. Personally, I don't think you need to blow a bunch of money on pricey yoga classes. I recommend just buying a mat and following along with free YouTube videos. My favourite yoga YouTube channel is "Yoga By Candace" and I highly recommend you check out her vast array of videos.

Chapter 6- Cardiovascular Training:

When you hear the word cardio please don't picture a treadmill. I never use treadmills and I think they are torture. My favorite form of cardio is swimming and I try to get into the pool at least twice a week. Swimming is difficult to get good at if you're a beginner, but once you get the hang of it, you'll never look back. In order to make swimming a good cardio workout you need cover a fair amount of distance in a workout. I aim for 1-2 kilometers per workout. Once you're able to relax in the pool and swim effortlessly, I find it to be a rather hypnotizing activity. I often swim for hundreds of meters without even realizing how far I've gone.

There's something about the quietness under the water that allows you to enter a kind of meditative state. I do some of my best thinking when I'm submerged in the pool doing a workout. The best way to get better at swimming (focus on front crawl) is to watch online technique videos, then get somebody to take a video of you swimming so you can compare techniques. Also, do lots of flutter kick and lots of strokes with a pull buoy to isolate different aspects of your stroke. Understanding how to coordinate your arms with your legs is difficult to do; I try to kick three times for every stroke I take. As far as breathing goes I try to breathe every 2 strokes, then 3 and then 2 so that the side I breathe on is being alternated.

Running is obviously what most people view as the epitome of cardio. Many people find running boring but that's likely because they're not having fun with it. I find trail running to be very fun and I also think running on the street is fun if you challenge yourself. I like to use a GPS and measure the distance of my runs, whether it's a 2km, 6km or 10km run, etc. Once I have a variety of different distances, I time myself and try to improve my time in all distances. Striving to better your times when you run is very rewarding and learning how to compete with yourself is crucial if you're usually working out on your own.

As far as running goes, the book "Born to Run" by Christopher McDougall has some great information in it. McDougall observes the behavior of elite Mexican running tribes and essentially finds that the key to running injury free is to keep your weight on your toes and not to slam down onto the overly cushioned heels of the running shoes. He also suggests implementing some barefoot running in order to force you to run on the balls of your feet and to strengthen your feet, which are always pampered by shoes. I followed these two tips and within days my lower back running pain was eliminated and I took my 10km time down from 41:11 to 38:57.

McDougall also looks into the benefits of chia seeds. He finds that one of the keys to the Mexican runners dominance, is the fact that they eat chia seeds for quick energy during their runs. I now mix chia seeds into my water when I run. The seeds are flavorless with a subtle texture and an amazing source of protein and omega 3's. I can genuinely say that I do feel more energized when I drink these seeds when I run and I recommend trying them.

More than any aspect of fitness, I find that cardio is the main branch for improving the way your body feels in general. When I have been running a lot I almost feel as though the resistance of gravity has been slightly decreased. I feel more spring in my step; I can get around faster, float up staircases and never seem to get fatigued in day-to-day life.

The feeling of having good cardio is spectacular, and the endorphin rush you feel after completing a good workout is fantastic. Don't get caught in the mind-set that cardio needs to be an extremely time consuming activity. While I do enjoy long cardio workouts, I often cut them back to 20-30 minutes if I'm on a time constraint. Cardio and functional strength workouts compliment each other nicely. If you're doing something like kettle bells or a weight circuit for a long time, make no mistake that you are also getting in a great cardio workout.

Chapter 7- Functional Strength:

Functional strength is the kind of strength that will aid you in your day-to-day tasks. Examples are; lifting and moving heavy objects, completing tasks without losing as much energy and just having more all-around full body strength. If you have a lot of functional strength you will feel more connected to your entire body and you will be able to operate as one complete unit. Instead of having strong legs but a weak back, or a powerful chest with a feeble core, functional strength will allow you to gain an overall sense of power throughout your entire body.

If you can bench press 300 pounds with proper form, that's good, but it doesn't necessarily mean you have functional strength. In the run of a day, how often do you have to lie horizontally and press weight completely vertically? Do you see my point? Functional strength will allow you to perform realistic tasks with minimal fatigue and maximum efficiency.

Enough talk, lets get down to some exercises that will give you functional strength. Kettle bells are the pinnacle of functional strength. Originating in Russia these awesome fitness tools have recently been popularized in North America. I bought a 40-pound kettle bell this year and it's the best fitness investment I've ever made. Some of my favorite kettle bell exercises are the two handed swing, snatch, upright row with squat, slingshot, halo and Turkish getup. As previously mentioned, if done correctly, kettle bells are a great functional strength and cardio workout. Even if you do a few sets- two minutes each for the exercises above, you will understand what I mean.

I find that the hanging pull-up and the burpee are two other gems of functional strength. By hanging pull-up I mean that there is no kip/swing involved, you're simply pulling your chin straight up over the bar. Focus on the quality of your reps, not the quantity. For burpees make sure you are getting your chest right down to the ground and jumping straight up at the end of each rep.

If you can increase your functional strength, then you will increase your everyday efficiency. When I first started building up my functional strength I primarily used a kettle bell. I was pretty worried that using a kettle bell, especially for swings, was going to hurt my already weak back. However, quite the opposite ended up happening. The more I worked out with my kettle bell, the more easily my body was able to perform as one functional unit. My back ended up getting stronger than it ever had been before because I learned how to use it functionally. When your functional strength increases you will know it because your entire body will feel different. It will be as though you just got some kind of a super power; you will feel lighter, stronger and faster.

Chapter 8- Sex:

Being a qualified sex expert I will attempt to……

No, that's a lie. I have no great secrets; all I know is that there is no better post workout activity than sex, obviously. A big part of the reason that people want to be fit is so that they can attract a mate who will want to have sex with them regularly. I know this is all very mind blowing, but stay with me.

I can think of no greater reward for being fit than the fact that you will likely have more sex. A greater sense of wellbeing is clearly the best reward, but sex is part of that greater wellbeing!

The only real secret that I use while having sex is the way I breathe. By being able to control your breathing the whole way through, you enable yourself to last longer. I didn't believe this when I read it in "The Multi-Orgasmic Couple," but the next time I had sex I realized how frantic my breathing was as I neared the end of my session. I began to breathe in a slow steady pattern and I was able to control myself much better. As I practiced this breathing technique I continued to get better and better. It's harder than it sounds because during sex your breathing becomes very out of sync with the motion of your body, but it's easy after a while. Just remember to focus on diaphragmatic breathing (deep belly breathing) and keeping a slow steady breathing pattern (Abrams & Chia).

As I previously mentioned, Brazillian Jiu Jitsu is a great way to learn how to control your breathing as well. Not to mention that it also strengthens your body in ways that are conducive to better, less fatigued sex.

Chapter 9- Mental Acuity:

Your brain is a tool and it must be worked constantly in order to stay strong. I don't feel 100% unless I've physically and mentally exerted myself. Read a book, watch some VICE news videos or have some meaningful, in depth conversations with friends. I think this last one is very important. If you only have friends who want to talk about getting drunk and the drama in their lives, maybe it's time to get some new ones. Every once in a while it's super refreshing to have deep conversations. Conversations about current events, the meaning of life, the universe or maybe the fact that we're all just on a rock, surviving because we are orbiting a massive fireball.

Never be afraid to look dumb or you will never learn. Ask questions until you find out exactly what you want to know. Your ego is your enemy; don't let it ruin you because once you stop learning, you become arrogant and irrelevant. Many of the habits mentioned in this book are designed to improve your mental acuity and I think you will really enjoy them.

Chapter 10- Morning Habits

Habit 1) Wakeup Call:

BUZZZZZZZZZZZZZZZZZ! Your alarm clock goes off. You're exhausted because you had a long day at work yesterday, but today is going to be different. Today is the first day you are going to practice the 30 ultimate habits that will revolutionize your life. So as soon as you hear that alarm clock go off I want you to jump out of bed immediately. Do not laze around trying to squeeze out a few extra minutes of sleep; it won't do you any good. In fact, if you don't get yourself up immediately and you spend 10- 15 minutes catching some last minute sporadic sleep, it is going to make you more tired during the first half of your day.

Once you hear that alarm it's time to cut your losses and accept the fact that you now have to face reality. The morning is a difficult but crucial time for a lot of people. If you have a rough morning, the rest of the day is sure to follow a similar pattern. But if you can manage to have a productive morning, the rest of the day will certainly be a productive one. So do not press that snooze button, just shut that alarm off and jump directly out of bed. If you need to do any thinking about the day ahead do it while standing or on your walk to the bathroom. This is going to sound painful, but **I recommend waking up 20-30 minutes earlier than you normally do.**

Habit 2) Drink Up:

Now that you're up and awake it's time to hydrate yourself as soon as possible, head into the kitchen and pour yourself a tall glass of fresh water. Cut up a lemon and squeeze a piece into your water then drop it in. Put the remainder of the lemon in a zip lock bag and stash it in the fridge for the next few mornings. Take a minute or two to drink this water and then poor yourself another glass to carry with you for the rest of the morning. Or you could just get yourself a big shaker bottle (BPA free) and fill that up from the get-go.

Drinking lemon infused water is a fantastic thing to do anytime of day, especially in the morning. Lemon water is a great antibacterial cleanser because it helps control unhealthy viruses and bacteria in your body. Lemon water will also reduce your levels of uric acid, which can lead to joint pain, as well as help your digestive system prepare for its first and most important meal of the day. Hydration is such a simple thing that so many people lack. Water is an amazing and vital resource that has become more and more unpopular due to things like coffee, tea, Gatorade, energy drinks, milk and juice. Water should be your priority fluid as it is one of the main building blocks of humanity, other liquids are peripheral!

Habit 3) Get Moving:

So far you should be about 5 minutes into your day so it's time to get your body moving immediately. A quick morning exercise routine is a very important habit to form. By getting yourself moving early in the morning you are saying to your body,

"Hey, this is what's going to happen. We're going to do a quick workout so that we can become energized once the endorphins get released. Get used to all of this movement because we are going to be going at this pace for the rest of the day!"

Getting your blood flowing will wake you up better than any amount of coffee ever could. I am the only person in my friend group who has never drank coffee in my life, even throughout a 5 year university program littered with late night studying and sleep deprivation. This amazes a lot of my friends and they ask me how I survived without coffee. Well, none of the people that ask me this question do a morning exercise routine, and that is the answer to their questions. I supplement the stimulating properties of caffeine with push-ups, burpees and squats. Here is the exercise set I normally do, depending on the amount of time I have on a given morning.

2 or 3 sets of: 5 burpees, 10 push ups, 15 squats.

You do not need to do these exact exercises and if you want learn some more detailed exercises and workouts, you will learn plenty more by the time you're finished reading this book!

Make sure you are hydrating during this workout and after it's complete. You shouldn't be totally exhausted once these exercises are done, they are not meant to be very strenuous. You just want to put in a good five or ten minutes of movement to get your heart rate up.

Fun fact: Richard Bronson has been quoted saying that the reason his productivity level is so amazingly high is all due to the fact that he works out on a daily basis. He said that if someone wants to be more successful in any aspect of their life, they must workout.

Habit 4) Loose Goose:

Stretching time. Once you complete your quick workout, before you eat it is time to do a quick stretching session. Do your favourite yoga routine or look online to find stretches for different body parts. I recommend stretching the following areas: Your legs, groin, lower back, chest, neck and triceps. By stretching you enable your body to become more loose and flexible. I recommend stretching after every workout, not extensively after a short workout like the one you just completed, but at least a little bit.

Using a foam roller is almost the equivalent of getting a decent massage. These rollers are great for the back, legs, glutes and hips. If your job requires you to sit for the entire day, then this habit is very important for you. Being sedentary for too long decreases flexibility at a rapid rate. The loss of flexibility is a sure-fire way to feel less energetic and more sluggish throughout the day.

Habit 5) Super Smoothie:

You must be starving at this point, so lets calm that craving. You've heard the saying before that breakfast is the most important meal of the day, and it is. You want the first meal that you deliver to your body to be nutritionally rich and packed full of foods that are conducive to giving you the energy that you deserve and need. Grab your blender and let's make a super smoothie.

Throw in 2 frozen bananas, 2 dates, half a cup of frozen blueberries, a handful of kale and spinach, ground flax seed, chia seeds, coconut water, unsweetened vanilla almond milk, half an apple, a spoonful of natural peanut butter, a teaspoon of matcha powder and a tablespoon of cinnamon.

The possibilities of smoothies you can make are virtually infinite. The above is simply one of my favorites and I guarantee after you drink it you will feel fantastic. The smoothie may not look appetizing in color but your body will thank you for drinking it, I promise. There are a ton of brain foods in this smoothie and there is no doubt that your mind and body will feel sharp after drinking it.

Habit 6) Extra Eating:

Some mornings my smoothie is not enough to hold me over, so I need to eat something else. If you feel the same way, I recommend some of the following:

-A couple scrambled eggs

-A banana with some natural peanut butter spread on it

-An avocado spread on light crackers

-A bowl of quinoa with cinnamon, pecans and almond milk added in

- Whole grain toast with coconut oil spread on it

- A plate of greasy nachos (just kidding, I'm just making sure you're still paying attention).

- A bowl of steel cut oats with cinnamon, walnuts and almond milk (maybe a touch of pure maple syrup)

Habit 7) Vitamin Fix:

With breakfast I like to take 500mg of vitamin C, 1000 IU of vitamin D, one Jamieson Vita-vim multivitamin, 1200mg of fish oil, and 1200 mcg of vitamin B12. Speak to a doctor or nutritionist before taking any of these supplements, but I do not foresee them being an issue. I like to ensure that my body gets all of its necessary nutrients before heading off to tackle my day. That being said, there are literally tons of other vitamins and supplements you can experiment with. It's really just all about finding what makes you feel the best on a day-to-day basis.

I find vitamin C significantly boosts my immune system and the only two times I have been sick in the past 6 years is when I neglected to take my vitamin C. Vitamin D is great because it provides you with the nutrients normally delivered to your body via the sun. I mostly take vitamin D during the cold Canadian winters. Multivitamins provide you with a myriad of different things (depending on the brand), all of which are fantastic for your body. Fish oils provide your body with essential omega 3 fatty acids, which help out with joint lubrication and brain function. Vitamin B12 helps with normal brain and nervous system function.

Habit 8) Ice, Ice Baby:

The short workout is complete, you're well fed and it is time to shower. Take the idea of a nice long, relaxing shower and throw it out the window. This shower is going to make our minds alert, our bodies fit and have us feeling completely replenished.

Get into the shower, just as you normally would. Do your usual routine and then prepare for something drastically different. Step outside of the warm water and turn the water as cold as it will go. Step back into the stream and let the ice-cold water run down the back of your neck. This will be uncomfortable and you will likely jump around a bit. This is a mental challenge more so than a physical one. Do not give in to your urge to jump out of the shower, or turn the water warm. Let the cold water hit every part of your body, control your breathing and try not to let yourself start sucking an excessive amount of air. You will feel a shortness of breath, but you need to keep telling yourself that everything will be ok. Your bodies natural reaction to freezing water is panic, because obviously if you are exposed to freezing cold water for too long, your body will start shutting down. Don't worry; you only need to stay under the water for three to five minutes (try for five!).

Once your watch tells you five minutes are up, you can turn the water warm again for ten seconds in order to regulate your body temperature, and then hop out of the shower. Who needs coffee right? If the workout didn't wake you up, this will wake you up like a kick to the teeth. Cold showering is not an easy thing to do, but the benefits of them are miraculous. Your mind will be extremely alert, your hair and skin will feel fresher than ever, your circulation will be top notch, your muscles will feel rejuvenated, since you literally just shocked your body and convinced it that it might be dying soon, your instinctual priority list has shifted completely. Survival instincts tend to flush out any peripheral thoughts that are not vital to that particular moment, meaning that you will feel less stressed and more relaxed.

Hopefully I have given you enough reasons to subject your body to the pains and chills of cold showering. Please don't knock it until you try it, seriously, it works wonders and everyone I know who has tried it is now addicted.

Habit 9) Self Motivation:

Once you step outside that shower and dry off, after you brush those fangs and check yourself out in the mirror, I want you to stare deeply at your reflection. Take a moment to appreciate the opportunity you have been given to live out your current day. Reflect on the fact that just you being here, alive on this planet, is the ultimate lottery victory with odds so incomprehensibly slim that your mind can't even begin to fathom them. One hiccup in the past, one wrong decision by your mother or father, or their mother or father, or their mother or father and you would cease to exist. The air we breathe right down to the earth we stand on is a complete miracle. Are you going to waste this miracle? Are you going to, even for one second, take this miracle for granted? No, you wouldn't even think about being complacent in this gift we call life. You're going to go about your day with unprecedented zeal and energy. You're going to attack this day with a burning fury. Your body is a complex machine and if any of its vital parts decides to quit, consciousness as you know it will be gone forever.

A lot of people will tell you to live every day like it's your last, but not me. I know that my last day on earth would not be one that I'd be very proud of. It would probably consist of skydiving, riding motorcycles WAY too fast and just so, so, so much sex. I want you to live every day in gracious way. Be appreciative of the things you have and do not dwell on things you do not. Attack every day with a passionate attitude and live every day like it's your very first day alive. Live it like you just sucked your first breath of fresh air after almost drowning in the ocean. Live it like you died and came back for a final chance at success!

Habit 10) Put it on Paper:

Take out a piece of paper or your phone and make a checklist. This checklist will aid you in completing all of your daily tasks/goals. Checklists are a great way to hold yourself accountable, and they allow you to feel accomplished when you draw that beautiful check mark on the page. By breaking your day down into a visible format, it allows your brain to better comprehend what you need to do and you will subconsciously begin planning out the steps you must take to in order accomplish everything on your list. Normally the difference between successful people and unsuccessful people is procrastination. By having a written list in front of your face, I find it becomes much more difficult to procrastinate.

While you're at it you should also take the time to write down goals. These could be financial goals, career goals, relationship goals, fitness goals, or anything you want. Write weekly goals, monthly goals, yearly goals, 5 year goals and even ten year goals.

Habit 11) Fill Up With an Extra Kick:

Now it's time to head off to work, school, the gym or wherever you must go today. Before leaving you should fill up a large water bottle with ice water and a teaspoon of chia seeds. If you have a transparent water bottle people might ask you if you are consuming frog eggs. These seeds are tasteless and you can drink them with ease. They will provide you with energy throughout the day by giving your body intermittent doses of omega 3 fatty acids, high quality protein and a ton of antioxidants. There are very few calories in chia seeds, meaning they have a very high cost-benefit ratio when it comes to calorie intake. You get a lot without having to consume a ton.

Chapter 11: Afternoon Habits

Habit 12) Rock Your Body:

Workout! You can do this wherever it fits into your schedule. Right now if you're saying to yourself "but I already worked out when I woke up," You did not. What you did was a brief exercise set to get your blood pumping to ensure that your body was awake. A real workout is a lot more extensive and it will require a bit more time. I will provide some brief examples of workouts that you could do during the day, most of which do not require a gym, or any kind of equipment for that matter.

A) 15-minute walk/ run.

- 3x10 reps of:

Pushups*, bodyweight squats, sit ups.

B) 3 sets of 1 minute of each exercise:

- jumping jacks, mountain climbers, burpees, flexed arm hang, reverse crunches, squats (rest 3 minutes between sets).

C) 1 x 1 minute on, 1 minute off, 1 minute on of each exercise: squat jumps, plank, burpees, flutter kicks, kettle bell swings.

D) 6 x 1 minute sprint run, 1 minute walk.

E) 30 minute jog, every 5 minutes perform 3 burpees and 15 squats (stop the time when you do these exercises then resume jogging).

Some of this terminology may be confusing to you. Fear not, you can find all of this information online or in the book itself. If all else fails you can contact me directly by email at:

johnmayo@hotmail.com

Try your best to make your workouts fun! Make sure you are constantly changing up your exercise routine because your body adapts very fast and you must keep it guessing. Track your progress and keep a workout journal so you can see how far you've come.

Hold yourself accountable to your workout schedule with an incentive system. If you miss a workout, then add an extra set to your next workout, or add another mile onto your next run. Alternatively, if you are consistently following your workout schedule, make sure you give yourself relaxing rest days and allow yourself to eat some 'cheat foods' every now and again.

Habit 13) Don't Waste Your Downtime:

Listen to good information, not repetitive music. If you have a long commute to work or wherever your day takes you, listen to audio books or podcasts. Instead of listening to "Shake It Off" for the 6th time in a row, give Taylor Swift a rest and listen to something educational and inspiring. There are tons of great audio books out there and even more fantastic podcasts. You can find a podcast on any topic you want, subscribe for free on iTunes and listen at your own leisure. The last job I worked was at a grocery store and the only thing that kept me sane was listening to motivational podcasts, namely, "The Joe Rogan Experience," which I highly recommend to everybody.

Habit 14) Positivity:

Realize that your thoughts truly do impact your reality. I'm not promoting the book "The Secret," in fact one of my favorite quotes about this book was said by comedian Dave Chappelle:

"This book tells people that the secret to life is positive imagery, try flying to Africa and telling those starving children that shit. All you have to do is visualize some roast beef, taters and gravy. The problem is; you have a bad attitude about starving to death."

Obviously there is nothing funny about children starving in Africa, but Chappelle uses his comedic wit to make a really good point here. You cannot, as "The Secret" teaches, will things into existence with positive thinking and imagery. Thoughts do impact reality a lot, but not to the extent that this book would lead you to believe - and yes, I have read this book cover-to-cover. You need to keep a positive mindset no matter what. Negative thinking only leads to more negative thinking, thus more negative results. Positive thinking leads to positive outcomes and thus more positive results. Both mindsets are cyclical; the latter is just a lot more beneficial than the other.

Habit 15) S-T-O-P

I know the statement 'stay positive' is very broad but I believe the key to positive thinking is altering your internal dialogue. If you always have negative thoughts bouncing around in your head, it's time you change that. You must learn to talk to yourself in a positive manner. I know this sounds very corny and believe me, when I was first told to do this, I laughed. But it really can make a massive difference in the way you conduct yourself and the way others see you. Some of the nicest people I know are also the most self-deprecating people I have ever met. Sometimes it is necessary that you are critical of yourself, your actions or a decision you made, but it is not healthy to never give yourself positive feedback. I find women are especially bad at giving themselves the credit they deserve.

During the day I want you to follow this simple acronym any time you are feeling down about something in your life.

S-T-O-P: Sit, Think, Objectify, Positivity

Take a seat somewhere that you can be alone for a few minutes. Think about what's on your mind, or whatever is troubling you at that moment. Be objective and try to look at the issue or decision, free of bias, from a neutral third party standpoint. Look at all of the positive aspects of whatever it is that is troubling you.

I love how good my girlfriend is at following the S-T-O-P acronym. Whenever we're together and something doesn't work out, I usually get frustrated, but she can always manage to STOP and throw a positive spin on almost anything that is going wrong. With her help I am really beginning to master the S-T-O-P method, and I find it to be extremely helpful.

Habit 16) Live in the Now:

"The now is here, the past is gone and the future will be nothing if the now is wrong." I made this quote up a few years ago when I was struggling financially. The message is that you must live in the now. Dwelling on the past or future too much is completely pointless. Sometimes in life you are going to have to feel out of control, and that's fine. You must train yourself not to panic and to only worry about the things that you can control on that given day. The more in the now you can live, the happier you will be.

I am constantly trying to minimize the time frame that I concern myself with. You can start big and then keep shrinking your time frame like I did. Let me explain; I began by forcing myself to only worry about the week in front of me. I eventually shrunk that down to a few days and before I knew it I was down to one single day. It felt great to only think about one day at a time and I noticed a jump in my productivity levels. I am currently working on cutting my time frame down to an hourly level, but that requires more practice.

Obviously I am not telling you to completely ignore events that are coming up in your future, or to not learn from mistakes you have made in your past. All I'm saying is that once you gain the information you need from past or future events, it's time to let them go and not dwell on them. Do not beat a dead horse, let the past be the past and welcome the future when it comes.

Habit 17) Be Selfish Sometimes:

Keep yourself motivated. This is certainly easier than it sounds, but by adopting the proper mind state, staying motivated can be very easy.

"I don't have to prove anything to anyone, I only have to follow my heart and concentrate on what I want to say to the world. I run my world"

-Beyonce

Beyonce Knowles just might be the most motivated female on the planet. Did you know while she was acting on a movie once that she was so determined to play her role perfectly, that she forgot to eat for two days? This woman is a true inspiration and I don't know many people, male or female, that have anything negative to say about her.

Keeping yourself motivated on a daily basis can be tiresome but you must always keep your goals at the front of your mind. By always reminding yourself of your daily goals, it allows you to persevere through whatever obstacles you may face. This is why in the earlier habits I told you to write your goals down so that you could physically see them on the paper. When it comes to completing your goals, being selfish is okay. Make sure you get your own stuff done before you start spreading yourself thin in an attempt to please others. It's like when your on a plane and the announcement comes on that says,

"If the cabin pressure changes drastically, an oxygen mask will deploy from above your head. Please safely secure your own mask before helping others with theirs."

They say this because if you try to help others before you help yourself, you may pass out, then two people are in trouble instead of just one. You are better able to help others once you help yourself first, never forget that and do not feel that being selfish is always a bad thing.

"I attribute my success to this: I never gave or took any excuse."

-Florence Nightingale

Habit 18) Role Models:

Surround yourself with motivated, inspirational and positive people. If you only have friends that put your dreams down, over-criticize you, or flake out on plans on a regular basis, then maybe it's time to get some new ones. Many people will do virtual Facebook friend cleanses, whereby they remove people that they no longer have a need for off of their friends list. Why don't more people do friend cleanses in real life?

I know tons of people that have that one friend from elementary school that constantly drags them down. Those friends who can just never seem to dig themselves out of a rut, and they constantly drag others into that rut with them. Just because you have been friends with someone for a long time, does not mean you have a forced life sentence of friendship to serve. Removing stress from your life requires you to remove stressors. If you have people in your life that are stressors, you need to minimize the time you spend with them, so as to minimize your own stress levels.

This may seem like a daunting task and it's true that cutting ties with people is much more difficult in the technologically advanced age that we live in. Learning to tell people no is an important skill to develop and by saying no to being friends with negative people, you will better develop this vital skill.

Habit 19) Limiting Stress:

If you're finding that you cannot remove particular stressful people from your life i.e., your boss, coworkers, family members etc. Then you must learn how to limit the amount of stress that they are putting upon you. One way to do this is to keep them content. If somebody is frustrating you, you must learn to control your emotions. Take some deep breathes and let's go back to the S-T-O-P method. Ask yourself if you are being reasonable. Take a minute to reflect on the particular person that is creating the problem for you. Think of one positive thing about the person. I know this sounds childish and silly but it allows you to calm your frustrations.

Even the most annoying people on earth have positive aspects to their personalities, whether it is tenacity, boldness, dedication, zeal, enthusiasm, punctuality, or a sense of humor. Once you have identified something positive that they bring to the table you will be able view the situation with a more unbiased lens.

There will be times where people in your life act in totally evil and irrational ways. During these times you will have to take a different course of action. If somebody starts yelling at me, or taking out his or her anger on me, I try to remain as calm as I can. By remaining calm you force the other person to feel foolish and embarrassed. These feelings will cause them to reevaluate what they're doing and potentially back down from the confrontation. Just think; fire (anger) is aggressive and sporadic, if you mix fire with fire you will only produce a larger flame.

Water (passivity) is calm and soothing, if you mix water with fire you can put out a potential inferno.

Habit 20) Nap Time:

Sometime during the day, if possible, take a twenty-minute nap. I know this won't suit everyone's lifestyle, but if you can fit it in, then you definitely should. Twenty minutes has been proven to be the optimal napping time. If you nap for too long, you will feel even more sluggish than you did before. This is because your body thinks that it is bedtime, so it begins to enter a deeper level of sleep. Twenty minutes is just long enough to give you a good shot of energy during your day- and trust me it works very well.

Chapter 12: Evening Habits

Habit 21) Snack Time:

Have a quick snack directly following your nap. By having a little snack now, you will reduce the amount you need to eat at dinner in order to feel full. Overeating is never a good thing and it's clearly no way to lose weight. Make sure the snack is not significant, perhaps a Clif bar or a banana dipped in natural peanut butter. If you have too big of a snack, you will stretch your stomach out and at dinner you will eat like a beast. Trust me, I've done it.

Habit 22) Walk it Off:

Once you get home from your long day of doing whatever it is that you do, I advise you take a short walk to blow off some steam. You don't have to walk for too long, I'd say 10-15 minutes at minimum. During this short walk you should reflect on the day that you just had. Determine whether or not you have accomplished all of the goals that you set for the day. If the day didn't go well, think about what you can do during the evening to make it better. If the day went well, then momentum is on your side and you should have no problem having a productive evening. Walking in the evening is also a fantastic idea so that you can get some exercise before eating dinner.

Habit 23) Read a Book:

Catch up on some reading. Reading is great, mind stimulating activity. It keeps your brain sharp and it is something that you should do every single day. Let your mind wander off into the different realms of the books that you indulge in. Studies show that reading helps to reduce stress, by removing your thoughts from your life and focusing them upon the words on the page.

Habit 24) Kill the Distractions and Meditate:

Turn your phone to airplane mode, shut off the television, walk away from the computer and begin to meditate in a quiet location. If you do not know how to meditate, you have infinite resources on the Internet- from YouTube to books and articles. Meditating obviously helps to reduce stress if done properly. The goal is to let go of any thoughts, positive or negative. Let your mind enter a state of emptiness where there is no concern or emotion. If you can get to this relaxed state, you will get a massive body high once you finish meditating. I never understood meditation until I experienced the amazing natural high that is associated with it. Now I try to meditate at least once a day.

Habit 25) Healthy Eating:

It's time for a delicious healthy dinner. Here are some healthy dinner selections that I like to eat often.

A) Mango avocado salad. I use one mango and avocado, cut them up and add black beans, lettuce, jalapeños, quinoa, salsa and low fat corn chips.

B) Mini pita pizzas. Add some pesto to pita bread with tomatoes, red pepper, onions and cheese. Bake the pita by the oven by itself first, add everything else and then put it back in the oven until the cheese melts

C) Spaghetti squash cooked in the oven. I like to add crushed tomatoes or a little bit of pesto.

Eating a healthy dinner is vital if you want to keep/get a good figure. It's amazing what a difference cutting unhealthy foods out of your diet can make in your life. When cooking anything in a pan I would advise that you use coconut oil instead of regular cooking oil or butter. Coconut oil is a truly amazing saturated fat and the health benefits of it seem to be limitless. Coconut oil is great for the skin and it can even help you lose weight if consumed in moderation. It is fairly dense and it will help to fill your stomach so that you don't need to fill it with unhealthy fats.

Habit 26) Lose the Bad Food:

It's fine to eat some unhealthy food from time to time, let's be honest; we all do it. But since a lot of us cannot control ourselves (myself included) it's best to keep unhealthy food out of our living environment all together. If it's not there you can't eat it and if all you've got is healthy foods, well you either eat that or you starve. DON'T BUY CRAP!

Habit 27) Make a List:

If you want to take some time off of your morning routine you could use your downtime in the evening to write your goal list for the following day. Writing goals in the morning may be stressful if you are on a time crunch. If you have the time in the evening, I recommend writing your daily goals for the following day, so you can really put in the necessary thought that this activity deserves. As I stated earlier, the more you make your goals physically visible, the more productive and successful you will be.

Habit 28) No More Food:

Do not eat ANYTHING after 9:00pm. Eating soon before bedtime results in unnecessary weight gain. This is an easy habit to get into, simply set an alarm on your phone for 9:00pm. Once that alarm goes off you can either grab one last quick snack, or you can stop eating for the remainder of the night. Consuming food before you sleep means that you have excess calories that cannot be expended because you are motionless in bed. You need to make sure that the calories you put in your body have the chance to get burned off before you sleep.

Habit 29) Daily Reflection and Stretch:

It's almost time for bed but we've got a few more things to do yet. During your night-time ritual of teeth brushing, face washing and all of that good stuff take a minute to reflect. Look at yourself in the mirror just as you did in the morning and smile. Hold that smile until it becomes awkward and give yourself credit for everything you got done. Head into your bedroom, but before jumping into your comfortable bed, pause. Reach your hands up into the air as high as you can and get onto your tippy toes. Stretch your entire body out and hold this position for as long as you can. After you can't hold the stretch any longer I want you to perform 10 squats (try to keep your legs parallel and get your bum right down to the floor. Keep your arms directly in front of you). Perform this stretch/squat set three times for a total of 30 squats.

This brief exercise set will not only tone your bum a bit (if done every night), but it will also help you sleep better. By slightly exerting your body before bed you will allow for better digestion of your dinner and a small fatigue of your muscles will help you drift off to sleep very quickly.

Habit 30) Set a Decent Bedtime

Make sure you are getting to bed at a decent time. Aim to get 6-8 hours of sleep every night. If you don't get yourself into a consistent sleeping pattern, then you will never be at your best. If for some reason you have to cut your sleep time down, try to add an extra 20-minute nap the following day, so that you can re-energize. Sleep is obviously vital for both mental and physical health, so ensure that you get proper amount or else you will be feeling stressed and fatigued the following day.

Chapter 13- 30 Days of Working Out at Home:

I encourage you to do one of these workouts per day for the next 30 days. You've got nothing to lose and absolutely no excuse since there is no gym required. I also encourage you to record your workouts so that once you complete them you can jot down some simple notes about how the workout went. As promised, there is no gym needed for any of the workout listed below. The most equipment you will need is a kettle bell/ dumbbell, a skipping rope and a chin-up bar. Before diving into the workout it will be important to know the key exercises so let's get started:

Explanation of Key Exercises:

Here I will be explaining all of the exercises that you will have to do in the 30-day program. I will do my best to explain them all but if any of them seem unclear there are certainly YouTube videos out there that can give you a more in-depth idea on how to do particular exercises.

Understanding Workout Terminology:

When reading a workout the first number is the number of sets and the second number is the number of repetitions per set. So if you see 4 x 20, that means four sets of twenty reps per set. During a set you perform every exercise in order with no rest between exercises unless otherwise instructed. Some workouts will be timed such as 3 x 1:00,

1:00 off, 1:30 on. For this workout you would be doing each exercise in the set for one minute, resting for one minute and then doing that same exercise for one and a half minutes.

The Pushup:

Your stomach should be flat on the ground. Keep your arms at shoulder width apart, keep your back straight and make sure your chest touches the ground at the bottom and that your arms are straight at the end of every repetition.

The Kettle Bell Swing:

You can use dumbbells instead of kettle bells; it's just a little harder to hold onto them. Remember to start light, grip the kettle bell with two hands, let it swing between your legs, slightly bend your knees, then thrust your hips and straighten your legs while keeping your back straight to swing the kettle bell up to eye level. Arms should be slightly bent, feet at shoulder width apart. The weight you use is totally dependent on the number of repetitions you will be doing. If you are a beginner I recommend starting with 20-25 lbs. Your arms should not be doing much work at all, they are simply holding and guiding the kettle bell, the power of your swing should be coming from your legs, hips, core and back.

The Burpee:

Start in the standing position, jump down until your chest is on the ground, do a pushup keeping your back flat, jump your legs up into a squatted position and spring yourself up into the air with your arms reaching to the sky. With practice this movement will become fluid, but it remains a very challenging exercise.

The Squat:

Squats should be performed with your feet at shoulder width apart. Put your arms straight out in front of you and keep your back straight as you lower your bum to your ankles, keeping your legs parallel to one-another. Keep your back straight and keep your weight on your heels. Once you get as low as you can, use your legs to push yourself back up to the standing position, all the while keeping your back straight and your core tight. Stand up in an explosive movement and thrust your hips outwards.

Jump Rope/ Skipping:

Make sure the skipping rope is the proper length. You can check this by holding the rope out in front of you, stepping on it with one foot and ensuring that the base of the handles comes up to at least your nipples. You can skip in a stationary position, or you can move around while skipping. Once you get good you can do some double unders (rope goes under you twice per jump), fast skipping, one leg skipping, heel skipping or side-to-side skipping.

The Pull-Up

Strict pull-ups are done straight up and down with your palms facing away from you. Do not swing or kip, you want to minimize the momentum and maximize the difficulty. I want you to only do strict pull-ups from now on. Get assistance if necessary when you're starting off, either from another person or by utilizing a weighted assistance mechanism found on certain pull-up machines.

The Mountain Climber:

Mountain climbers are great for your core. To perform, hover above the ground keeping your body horizontal. You should be on your toes and hands with your arms straight. One at a time, bring your knees towards your chest in an alternating motion. Every time both legs go in and out, you have completed one repetition.

Leg Lifts:

For leg lifts you want to lie flat on your back with your legs completely straight. Bring your legs up from the ground until they are at 90 degrees relative to your torso and then lower them until they hover above the ground. During the exercise you can either have your hands on the floor, or under your bum if you're finding the exercise difficult.

Squat Jumps:

Squat jumps are performed just like a regular squat, but you jump into the air about 1 foot upon extension of the legs.

Flexed Arm Hang (F.A.H):

Flexed arm hang is when you hang onto a chin-up bar with your arms bent and your eyes level with the bar. Stay up as long as the specified time says and if you lose your grip get right back up. This is a very difficult exercise.

The Reverse Crunch:

Reverse crunches are performed by lying flat on your back with your hands on the ground beside you. Your legs should be bent with your feet on the ground and you simply bring your knees up towards your chest and then back down to perform one repetition.

The Russian Twist:

For a Russian twist, sit down, lean back and let your legs hover above the ground. Rotate your core around side to side with your hands in front of you and your chest up. Let your hands touch the ground on either side of you to complete one full rep.

The Burpee Pull-Up

Burpee pull-ups are just like regular burpees, except for that when you jump up you need to grab a bar and do a pull-up at the end to complete a full rep. Use the momentum of your jump to assist you in your pull-up. You may find it easier to do the pull-up with one hand gripping the bar with your palm facing out, and one hand with the palm facing in.

The Plank:

For a plank you want your stomach facing the ground. Put your elbows underneath your shoulders and lift yourself off the ground. Your weight should be on your elbows and your toes. Try to keep your back perfectly flat (don't sag your hips down to the ground or lift your bum really high into the air). Keep your abs tight and ensure that you have a comfortable base on your elbows/ forearms.

Leg Ins:

Leg ins are done from the plank position. Once in position, bring your right knee to your right elbow, and then back. Do the same with your left side and that equates to two reps.

Pikes:

Pikes are also done from the plank position. Simply arch your back and stick your bum into the air, returning to the plank position to complete one repetition.

Flutter Kicks:

For flutter kicks you must lie on your back. Hover your legs above the ground and move them up and down as if you were kicking in the water. Up and down on each leg is one repetition.

U-Sits:

Sit on your bum with your knees bent and your feet hovering about one foot off the ground. The starting position for this exercise requires your legs to be straight (feet still hovering) and your arms should be straight, but off to the side as if you were trying to stop the walls from crushing in against you. To complete one repetition you must bend your knees up into your chest and clap your hands (arms remaining straight) in front of your knees.

The Super Burpee:

I want you to think 1 sit-up, 1 pushup, 1 burpee. I have dubbed this the super burpee because it is a superb exercise. Try to make this as smooth of a movement as you can. Do one complete sit-up, roll over onto your stomach and do a push up and then jump straight up into the air, like you would at the end of a regular burpee.

The Lunge Walk:

One leg at a time, step one foot out in front of you as far as you can, while dropping the opposite knee down to the ground (don't actually touch the knee on the ground, but get as close as you can). Get a nice smooth walking pattern going as you continue to switch legs.

The Sit-Up With Twist:
Keep your feet flat on the ground, knees pointed up to the sky and your hands touching your ears. Once you have fully sat up I want you to touch your right elbow to your left knee and then your left elbow to your right knee. This gets your abs a little more involved than a regular sit-up does.

Wall Sits:

 Put your back flat against a wall, bend your legs at about 90 degrees and hover above the ground like you are sitting in an invisible chair. Hold the position for as long as the specified time says.

Leg Ups:

While holding onto a pull-up bar with your arms straight, bring your knees up to your chest and flex your abs.

Roll Back Burpee:

Jump straight up into the air, upon landing let yourself fall back onto your bum and roll onto your upper back like you're doing a reverse crunch. Roll back up onto your feet (using your arms to push of the ground if you need to) and then jump straight back up into he air.

Kettle Bell Thrusters:
Hold the kettle bell with both hands, squat with the kettle bell and upon extension of the legs press the kettle bell up over your head. Use the momentum of your squat to force the kettle bell upwards in one fluid motion.

Kettle Bell Squats:

Perform a squat while holding a kettle bell. Hold it however you feel comfortable, I prefer to hold it by the handle while keeping my arms straight, but you can also hold it by the horns and keep it close to your chest. If you really want a challenge you can hold it above your head with one hand.

High Knees:

Run on the spot with your knees coming up to your chest. Each time both legs go up and down you've done 1 rep

Kneeling Super Mans:

Start on your hands and knees. Reach your right arm out straight in front of you and extend your left leg behind you. Once extended bring your right elbow to your left knee. Do the same with your left arm and right leg to complete one rep.

Penguins:

Lie on your back with your legs bent, knees pointing towards the sky. Your arms should be straight by your side. Touch your left foot with your left hand and your right foot with your right hand to complete one rep. Tighten your abs and try to engage them as much as possible.

Plank Leg Lifts:

From the basic plank position alternately lift your legs up into the air. Lift both legs once to complete one rep

Speed Skaters:

Swing your left leg behind you (in a sort of sideways lunge) and touch your right foot with your right hand, then swing your right leg behind you and touch your left foot with your left hand to complete one rep.

Day 1:

Perform 6 sets of 20 squats. Between each set jump rope for 30 seconds.

*Rest 1 minute between sets

NOTES:
Skipping may prove slightly difficult after having done squats, but use this skipping time to shake your legs out and prepare for the next set of squats.

Day 2:

Warm up with a 20-minute jog, and then perform:

4 Sets of:

5:00 jump rope

1:00 F.A.H

30 kettle bell swings

* Rest 2:00 between sets

NOTES:
This workout will test your grip. After performing F.A.H and kettle bell swings your hands will be tired. Try to shake them out well during the 2 minutes of rest to prepare for the next set.

Day 3:

1-hour jog/walk

*No rest

NOTES:

The goal here is to not stop moving at all during the entire
hour. Try to run the whole time without stopping for rest!
ONLY WALK IF NECESSARY.

Day 4:

Run for 10 minutes and then do a 1-mile run for time.

NOTES:

If you don't want to run on a treadmill (which I recommend doing because running outside is awesome) then you can either buy a GPS watch or download a free app on your phone to help to track your distance. I use the app "RunKeeper" and I find it works really well. The reason I want you to time your 1-mile run is so that you can track your running progress during the next month. Try to do the run at a decent pace so that you're very tired at the end of it.

Day 5:

1 set of:

50 jumping jacks

50 jump rope

40 jumping jacks

40 jump rope

30 jumping jacks

30 jump rope

25 mountains climbers

20 reverse crunches

20 u-sits

10 burpees

10 leg overs

10 lunge walks

NOTES:

Don't rest at all during this workout, just do the entire set straight through. By not resting you get your cardiovascular system involved and it forces you to become more mentally resilient. Having a strong mind is essential to having a good workout because if your mind is unfocused or in a negative place you will have a really tough time completing difficult workouts.

Day 6:

4 sets of the following exercises:

10 burpees

20 pushups

30 squats

40 mountain climbers

50 jumping jacks

60 jump ropes

*Rest 20 seconds between exercises and 2:00 between sets.

NOTES:

You should find that each exercises gets easier and easier so try to keep the intensity high as your progress through the workout.

Day 7:

REST DAY

Go for a nice long 1-2 mile walk and give your whole body a good stretch afterwards. Rest days are very important as they give your body and muscles a good chance to recuperate and prepare for the week ahead.

CONGRATULATIONS for making it this far in the 30-day program! But don't stop here, you still have 13 tough days remaining, but with focus and determination you will succeed!

Day 8:

Jump rope for 8 minutes then in 10 minutes complete as many sets as possible of:

10 Pushups

10 Sit-ups with twist

10 Burpees or 10 pull-ups

*No rest, try to work hard for the entire 10 minutes set

NOTES: 1 set is 10 pushups, 10 sit ups with twist and 10 burpees or 10 pull-ups. Make sure you record your results so that you can compare results when we do this workout one more time at the end of the program. I have given you the choice between burpees and pull-ups; they are both very challenging exercises so there's no easy option, trust me!

Day 9:

Warm-up with a 10-minute jog and then do the following running set:

4 sets of:

1:00 jog

20 seconds sprint

2:00 jog

30 seconds sprint

3:00 jog

* No rest between the sprints and jogs. Rest 1 minute between sets.

NOTES:

Obviously you will need some sort of a stopwatch for this workout. This workout is good because it involves your cardiovascular system but it also forces you be explosive during the sprints by incorporating some anaerobic exercise.

Day 10:

5 sets of:

100 jump ropes (or 50 double unders if you are able)

20 burpees

10 Russian twists

NOTES:

The burpees will undoubtedly be the most challenging aspect of this workout. The key to a good burpee is being as smooth as possible on every single repetition. Don't allow your body to get out of control and don't let your posture fall apart. Stay in control and make every rep count.

Day 11:

Warm up with a 45-minute run and then do the following:

2 x 5 minutes of as many burpee pull-ups as possible.

*Rest 5 minutes between sets

NOTES:

This is going to be a tough one but you can do it! Use the 5 minutes of rest to rehydrate and don't allow your body to tense up during this time. Shake yourself off and keep yourself moving around. Try to remain consistent and get close to the same number of burpee pull-ups on each of the two 5 minute sets. This will be very challenging since you will already be tired on the 2nd set, but give it your best attempt!

Day 13:

Warm-up with a 10 minute jog and then perform the
following:

3 sets of:

20 squat jumps

30 walking lunges

40 jumping jacks

3 minute jog

*No rest between sets, use the jog at the end of each set as
your rest by controlling your breathing and keeping your
body moving.

Day 14:

REST DAY

Go for a minimum of a 3-mile walk. Once the walk is complete spend at least 30 minutes stretching out your entire body. If you don't have a foam roller I strongly recommend that you get one. Foam rollers are great to use after stretching as they really allow you to loosen up your muscles even further. I enjoy rolling out my back, quads, calf muscles, inner thighs, shins and lats.

Day 15:

Each main exercise is accompanied by an easier, alternate exercise. On the first set perform 1:00 of the main exercise and 1:30 of the alternate exercise. On the second set perform 1:30 of the main exercise and 1:00 of the alternate exercise.

Perform 2 sets of the following:

main: pushups, alt: seal jacks

main: roll back burpees, alt: reverse crunches

main: Kettle bell squats, alt: high knees

main: lunge walks, alt: jump rope

main: kettle bell thrusters, alt: leg lifts

main: double unders, alt: Russian twists

main: kettle bell swings, alt: kneeling super mans

main: leg ups, alt: speed skaters

*Rest 30 seconds between exercises and 6 minutes between sets

NOTES:

This workout may seem complex at first glance, but once you get into it you will find that it's not that difficult (as far as understanding it goes). The workout itself is definitely challenging and it takes a while. Getting through 2 sets of each exercise is going to be very draining, but once you complete it you will feel awesome about yourself!

Day 16:

Warm-up with a 20-minute jog then do:

3 sets of:

50 high knees

40 reverse crunches

30 leg ups

20 squat jumps

10 roll back burpees

5 burpee pull-ups

*Rest 20 seconds between exercises and 2 minutes between sets.

NOTES:

The exercises get harder as the reps decrease. Stay explosive and attack each exercise with intensity!

Day 17:

Warm-up with 10 minutes of jump rope then do:

4 X 15 reps of

kettle bell squats

kettle bell swings

kettle bell thrusters

*Rest 10 seconds between exercises and 1 minute between sets

NOTES:

Use a kettle bell/ dumbbell weight that is comfortable for you. I would use about 50 pounds for this workout but I'm a 185 pound male. I think a good weight for most females would be about 20 pounds.

Day 18:

Warm-up with a 10-minute jog, then perform 1 set of:

60 jump rope, 60 high knees

50 jump rope, 50 Russian twists

40 jump rope, 40 penguins

30 jump rope, 30 u-sits

20 jump rope, 20 leg ups

10 jump rope, 10 burpees

10 jumping jacks, 10 squat jumps

20 jumping jacks, 20 pikes

30 jumping jacks, 30 mountain climbers

40 jumping jacks, 40 leg ins

50 jumping jacks, 50 kneeling superman's

60 jumping jacks, 1-minute plank

*No rest! Use the jump rope as your rest

NOTES:

This seems like a complicated workout until you catch on to the simple pattern. Essentially you are doing a descending ladder, immediately followed by an ascending ladder. Stay focused and allow the jump rope sections to be your rest.

Day 19

Warm-up with a 1-mile jog then perform:

4 X (1:30 plank, 1:00 rest, 1:30 wall sit, 1:00 rest, 1:00 plank, 30 seconds rest, 1:00 wall sit)

*Rest 2:30 between sets

NOTES:

This workout will test your resolve. Grab a stopwatch and get it done. The time will go slower the more you think about it so try to focus on something other than the pain and the time. Allow your mind to drift as you push through this workout.

Day 20

Warm up with 3 X 15 reps of

Jumping jacks

High knees

Mountain climbers

Then perform:

10 X 50 seconds jog, 10 seconds sprint

*No rest!

10 X 40 seconds jog, 20 seconds sprint

*No rest!

10 X 30 seconds jog, 30 seconds sprint

*No rest!

*Rest for 2 minutes between sets

NOTES:

Do not stop moving during the rest in this workout. If you stop moving after sprinting your muscles are sure to cramp up and fail you. Use the jogging as your rest during the sets and ensure you are breathing in a controlled manner.

Day 21

REST DAY

Go for a nice long 1-2 mile walk and give your whole body a good stretch afterwards. Rest days are very important as they give your body and muscles a good chance to recuperate and prepare for the week ahead.

Only 9 days left until you've completed the program. Hopefully at this point working out has become a regular habit and you are feeling fit and energized every single day. Keep going and never quit!

Day 22

Run 20 minutes out, and then perform 30 squats, 20 mountain climbers and 10 burpees. Run 20 minutes back and then do 30 squats, 20 mountain climbers and 10 burpees.

*No rest.

NOTES:

You may find it challenging to run after completing a short workout set. The main thing to keep in mind is that you must control your breathing and not let yourself take panic breaths. Once you sacrifice your breathing you're sure to cramp up.

Day 23

Warm up with 15 minutes of jump rope, and then perform:

3 sets of:

10 kettle bell swings

10 seconds rest

20 kettle bell swings

20 seconds rest

30 kettle bell swings

30 seconds rest

40 kettle bell swings

40 seconds rest

ETC......

CONTINUE ADDING INCREMENTS OF 10 SWINGS
AND TEN SECONDS OF REST UNTIL YOU CAN'T
BUILD ANY HIGHER. ONCE YOU FAIL YOU HAVE
SUCCESSFULLY COMPLETED ONE SET.

NOTES:

Rest for 2 minutes after each set

Day 24

Warm-up with 100 jumping jacks and 100 high knees, then perform:

6 sets of:

1:00 jump rope, 30 seconds speed skipping, 2:00 jump rope, 1:00 speed skipping

*Rest for 2 minutes between sets.

NOTES:

If you can do double unders then you should do those instead of speed skipping.

Day 25

Warm-up with 3 minutes of jump rope then:

Perform 3 sets of the following:

100 jump ropes

3:00 plank

5 burpee pull-ups

10 kettle bell squats

30 kneeling supermans

5 roll back burpees

30 u-sits

5 super burpees

20 pushups

20 kettle bell swings

*Rest 20 seconds between exercises and 2:00 between sets

NOTES:

This will be a challenging and long workout, but you can do it!

Day 26

Run for 10 minutes and then do a 1-mile run for time.

NOTES:

Compare this run time to the one you did back on day 4 and see how much progress you've made!

Day 27

Warm-up with 2 minutes of jump rope, then do:

2 sets of:

1 Minute of each exercise:

Speed skaters

Burpees

Plank

kettle bell swings

leg over's

flexed arm hang (F.A.H)

penguins

mountain climbers

flutter kicks

*Rest 2 minutes between sets.

NOTES:

Do not rest between exercises. You should transition from one exercise to the next in as little time as possible. Plan your workout beforehand and ensure you have everything set up properly to allow for minimal transition times.

Day 28

REST DAY

Go for a nice long 1-2 mile walk and give your whole body a good stretch afterwards. Rest days are very important as they give your body and muscles a good chance to recuperate and prepare for the week ahead.

Only 2 days left until you've completed the program. Hopefully at this point working out has become a regular habit and you are feeling fit and energized every single day. Keep going and never quit!

Day 29

Jump rope for 8 minutes then In 10 minutes complete as many sets as possible of:

10 Pushups

10 Sit-ups with twist

10 Burpees or 10 pull-ups

*No rest, try to work hard for the entire 10 minutes set

NOTES: 1 set is 10 pushups, 10 sit ups with twist and 10 burpees or 10 pull-ups. Make sure you record your results so that you can compare results from the same workout back on day 8. How much progress have you made during the program?

Day 30

Warm-up with a 10-minute run, then do:

The Kamikaze:

4 Sets of:

20 burpees

30 kettle bell swings

10 pull ups

30 lunge walks

50 squats

1:30 plank

30 mountain climbers

20 U-sits

15 reverse crunches

20 Russian twists

*Rest 5:00 between sets

NOTES:

This is one of my favorite workouts and I've featured it in some of my other fitness books. The Kamikaze will offer you a full body blast. You will love to hate this workout! Enjoy.

Conclusion:

Great work on the workout program! In conclusion, this book is merely a representation of my own personal experiences and the guidelines I try to follow in order to become a more happy and productive person. Everything I said is exactly what I do, because it works very well for me, but this is not to say that it will work for you.

Modern life seems to trick our minds into thinking that "this is the way I should behave, sleep eight hours, work eight hours, eat when I can, have sex when I can, try to raise a family and repeat. This is the cycle that traps many people and before they know it they are unhappy with their lives, likely due to the fact that they are unhappy with themselves. Just because our species has evolved in exponential ways over a brief period of time, doesn't mean we can forget our roots and genetics.

Our species conquered due to our rapid evolution of intelligence and fitness. Remember, it's survival of the fittest, not the mere existence of the complacent. We are at the top of the food chain because we have the physical abilities to act upon our ideas.

It's a well-known fact that human beings are the best long distance runners on planet earth. Yes it's true that cheetahs could catch and eat us with ease. It would also not be wise to place a wager on a human at a horse race. Humans could however run down both of these animals over a long distance until their hearts exploded, the reason? Sweat! Humans are able to sweat and when this sweat evaporates, our overall body temperature is cooled.

Many people hate sweating but I embrace this vital trait. Sweat lets me know that I'm exerting myself in an effective way and burning calories. Imagine if primitive humans behaved in the ways that the average person behaves today. Lying around in caves, entertaining themselves with futile activities. We would have never made it out of that era and likely gone extinct if that was the case. The reason that didn't happen was all due to a lack of choice. There were no T.V.'s, cell phones, iPods or things like that; there were only the priorities of food, shelter, water and reproduction. If you weren't mentally and physically fit enough, you would perish, period.

Choice has quickly become societies enemy and has forever altered our priorities. Distractions have become so normalized that people forget what's important. It should be abundantly clear that we are not genetically designed to be sedentary all day. Your body doesn't release endorphins if you beat a video game or finish a season of Breaking Bad. Endorphins are released under moments of stress, pain (like repeated exercise), and extreme pleasure. I think of Endorphins as a natural reward for doing something that will increase your chances of survival. If sex didn't feel so damn good I guarantee we would have a less populated planet.

If you don't make time for physical activity in your life, you either will or currently are feeling the consequences. I think that if you trap and suppress your physical needs, your body has a tendency to "short circuit" and fulfill this physical need in other ways, such as violence or forced drama in your life. I wish I could do an experiment on every single person on earth who suffers from depression, or who is just generally unhappy. I bet a large majority of these people do not exercise and I bet that if they did a lot of them would throw their prescriptions out the window.

I'm not trying to discount mental illness in any way. There are a lot of people who desperately need medication in order to function, due to major chemical imbalances in their brains. My point is that in some cases, people's feelings of emotional imbalance could be fixed or ameliorated through greater levels of fitness.

Let's stop lying to ourselves, I mean who doesn't want to look into a mirror and say, "damn, I look great and all my hard work is paying off?" That's an awesome thing to desire and I think we all should. Break your monotonous cycle and make room for your own fitness. Not only will you look better, but I guarantee you will feel more mentally and physically balanced as well.

If I have a difficult decision to make in my life, if I'm frustrated about something or if I just need some moving meditation, I go for a run or a swim and it helps immensely.

I think there's something hypnotic about continuous movement. The ability to feel control over your entire body allows you to transfer this feeling of control to issues in your life.

This book will hopefully serve as your brief, yet difficult guide to a greater level of general fitness. Allow me to reiterate: Fitness is not a simple thing to achieve or maintain and anybody who tells you otherwise is lying to you, likely to make a quick buck off of you. Fitness must be achieved, maintained and constantly improved upon. It is a lifestyle choice that will make you a happier person. You only have one body, so why not make it the best physical specimen that you possibly can.

Pardon yet another car analogy but I find it ironic that some people spend their entire lives saving up for dream cars. They feel that if they can just afford that Ferrari, they will be a complete and happy person. People will go into debt to buy a nice car, yet throw their own personal well being on the back burner. Invest your money in something natural and real like your body, but keep in mind that fitness doesn't need to be expensive! I bet a woman would find a healthy guy in a Honda to be more attractive than a fat-ass in a Ferrari. On the other hand, who really knows what women want? All I know is that I'd rather feel good in my own body than in a luxury car, but I'm obviously going to strive to be fit and also drive a badass car.

These thirty daily habits and workouts will help you minimize stress, lose weight and remove negative thinking. Reading this book was not the important part. The important part comes next. Are you going to put this book down and go back to living life according to your usual routine? Are you going to say to yourself "that was a decent book, but it's far too complicated and tedious to apply to my busy life"? No you're not, do want to know why? You read this book to create a change in your life, a necessary change that you have been waiting to make.

You will make the time to incorporate these habits into your life and you will begin to feel the benefits of them. For the first few days you will be overwhelmed, but you will persevere. Once you engrain this daily routine into your lifestyle it will become automatic. You will no longer have to think about following the steps, you will naturally follow them and you will become fit, positive and way less stressed. I urge you incorporate these habits into your life and reap the benefits.

I look forward to hearing your success stories and I will be here every single step of the way. You can send me an email any time and I will be here to help you (johnmayo@hotmail.com). I hope you find the information in this book useful and applicable.

If you enjoyed the workouts in this book that incorporated kettle bells, then check out this awesome kettle bell channel on YouTube that delivers FREE awesome weekly kettle bell workouts:

Just search "Ladybells Fitness" on YouTube.

The ladies in these videos know how to deliver gruelling workouts that are also very well designed. I've done many of the workouts and they definitely have my stamp of approval!

DON'T FORGET MY FREE GIFT TO YOU:

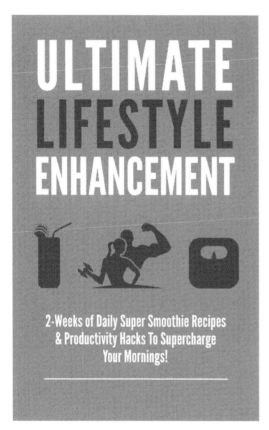

Type in the below link to get it for FREE right now

https://zenithpublishing.leadpages.net/lifestyle-enhancement/

Enjoy!

CHECK OUT ANOTHER ONE OF MY TITLES

If you enjoyed "Healthy Habits" I guarantee you will enjoy the title on the following page.

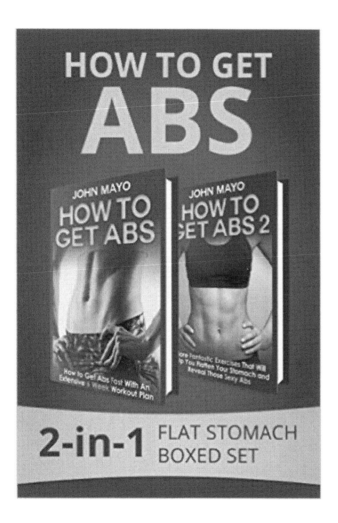

How To Get Abs: 2-in-1 Flat Stomach Boxed Set

How to Get Abs Fast With An Extensive 6-Week Workout Plan

John Mayo

Table of Contents:

1) Introduction:

If you don't have to work hard for something, then it's usually not worth getting!

We all know why you're here, so let's get right down to it. First things first, congratulations for taking it upon yourself to flatten out your stomach. Abs and a flat stomach are probably the most desired aspect of the human body for a lot of people. Human beings will put themselves through immense pain at the gym, just so they can feel good about themselves when they take off their shirts. Can you really blame these people though? Let's face it; abs and a flat stomach look great and it's completely understandable that people want to achieve this look.

So who am I and why should you care? I'm the guy who's going to help you achieve your fitness goals. I'm a guy who has had abs for almost his entire life. I'm not being cocky about it; it's just a fact. I have been an athlete for my entire life and fitness is something that I take very seriously. I am a kayaking coach in Nova Scotia, Canada, and my passion is helping people increase their fitness level. Since abs are a very sought after thing, I really enjoy helping people flatten their stomachs and get ripped abs.

Let me be honest though, abs are not easy to get, nor are they easy to maintain. Anything in life that is worthwhile takes hard work and dedication to achieve and getting abs is no different. I have a theory about abs; I think that one of the main things that make abs so sexy is that when people see a flat stomach or ripped abs, they understand the hard work and self-discipline associated with this achievement. I think a lot of people view a person's stomach as a direct reflection of their personality, so when somebody has no belly fat, people generally think of that person as dedicated, focused and determined. Unless of course they cheated and got liposuction. Perhaps you think this theory is a stretch, but I believe it to hold quite true for most people.

So what makes this fitness book different from all the other "get abs fast" books out there? One word, honesty. I will not lie to you and tell you that at the end of this 6-week program you will have the chiseled abs and flat stomach that you've always desired. But if you take the information, workout techniques and fitness strategies that I am going to provide to you in the following pages, apply them continuously and never give up, you will undoubtedly get the results that you desire.

Make no mistake; this is going to be a difficult task. I talk a lot in my other fitness books about forming good habits. One you make something a habit, it becomes automatic and easy. The less you have to think about making good, healthy choices, the better off your life will be. This is why it is very important to get into good fitness routines and stick with them! That's where I come in. I am very good at getting people into healthy routines and creating manageable programs that will better their health. This specific book is obviously going to focus on how to get abs and if you follow along and do not stray from my program, I can almost guarantee that you will see results.

Strap yourselves in, focus, tighten those abs up and let's get going!

Made in the USA
Las Vegas, NV
09 March 2024

86943888R00066